Lessons Learned

Lessons Learned

About Dementia

from My Mother

Help for Interacting with A Loved
One with Dementia/Alzheimer's

Sally Stap

Dedication

My mom used to say, "Enough is enough and I've had enough."

Contents

An Alternate Reality

"Of sound mind" is not a steady state.

Sharing life with a person suffering from dementia requires patience. Caregiving for a person who is living in an altered state existence requires a paradigm shift. Every person's path is different and leads through a new world entered with little guidance and fewer answers. A loved one, who has possibly been rock steady for life, has faltered and changed into a confused and sometimes defiant bully. Let us take a little journey from their perspective. I can only imagine what it would feel like to be seemingly transported in time to years into the past.

Consider these scenarios from the perspective of someone who is losing their memory:

"What I knew is now no longer within grasp. I remember being at home with my parents and siblings. Suddenly, I am being told they are all dead. I look in a mirror expecting to see a young person and I see an old, wrinkled and gray-haired stranger. I want to go to my room and go to bed. However, there is no familiar room anymore."

. . . .

"I can only describe the man who lives with me as a caregiver who my family must have hired to watch me. He wants to sleep in my private room at

night. He is always telling me to take pills I do not recognize and do not know what they might do to me. I ask him where my husband is, and he claims to be exactly that. I would know if he was my husband."

....

"A nice man comes to visit me and my husband one day and calls me Mom. I correct him and he is silent. He tells me stories about growing up as my son. I do not know this man. How can that be?"

....

"People claim they are laughing with me and not at me. All I did was give the lady's dog a biscuit. She claims I already gave him several in that same visit. I do not know why she is saying such a thing. I did not even know there were dog biscuits in the

cupboard until just now. To be polite, I laugh along but am sure the dog has not had a biscuit. He's looking at me with big brown eyes and looks eager and hungry."

I could continue, but these snapshots demonstrate that a person with dementia is not in our reality. We need to recognize and adapt our communication to better interact. If you recognize your loved one in any of these scenarios, you are not alone. Through examples, I will share some points to ponder and tips to consider for your interactions. First, I will cover some basic concepts.

Dementia Definition

Dementia is an umbrella term encompassing over one hundred conditions impairing memory and behavior. There are several common diseases, which can each be researched individually. I am not a professional so I will not go into detail, which you can find in many books and online. However, as a brief reference, the most common dementia diagnoses are:

Alzheimer's – degenerative disease that attacks the brain

Vascular Dementia - reduced blood flow

usually due to a stroke or mini-strokes

Parkinson's – a degenerative disorder

Lewy Body – a protein disorder in the brain

Frontotemporal Dementia - disorders affecting the frontal and temporal lobes

With the assistance of your physician, a proper diagnosis can be obtained, which will allow you to further research the specific variation of dementia your family is experiencing. When considering what is best for your loved one, keep in mind you are now dealing with a different person who is incapable of making major and even minor life decisions. Activities they previously loved to do may now be confusing or uncomfortable for them. As hard as it is, the person as you have always known them is gone and a new, changing one has taken their place. It may not be possible to include them in decision making about their care.

Sometimes we will never know exactly what or when things went off the rails. My mother descended into dementia that was never tested or formally diagnosed, other than clear observations by family confirmed by her physician. He generally referenced dementia or Alzheimer's disease. However, we did have suggestions by her cardiac physician that she may have had multiple mini strokes. So, being ready for a lot of uncertainty is good preparation. Take it a day at a time.

Medically, Urinary Tract Infections (UTIs)

can increase confusion and increase or mimic dementia. As the brain continues to deteriorate, the body will slowly lose the ability to do physical functions so eating becomes difficult. The loss of bowel control may happen, or you may find that your loved one repeatedly makes trips to the bathroom, but you learn that nothing has been happening in there. It is hard to track physically what is happening. Become informed and find a support group online or in your community if possible.

A Conversation

Confusing and frustrating, dementia is a diabolical disease. This scientifically identified disease alters minds and changes loved one's cell by cell, stripping away one memory at a time. Dementia re-shapes minds and glazes expressions before our eyes. With no known cure, we are helpless to do anything about it. Regardless of effort, love, or intent, it makes a wide swath through lives and minds.

Dementia is also mind-altering for the family. Here is a conversation I had with my mother one day shortly after moving her into a memory care facility:

"Hi, Mom. How are you today?"

Blank stare.

"Mom, it's me, your daughter."

"I know who you are. You put me in this prison."

"Mom, it's so nice to see you. It's a beautiful day." I tried to cheerfully redirect the mood.

"How's the family?"

"Everyone is doing well, Mom." Followed by giving her five minutes of updates about everyone in the family.

"Why am I here?"

"Mom, I love your picture of the Cross on the wall. I remember when you made that when we lived on the farm years ago."

"Who are you again? Are you my daughter or sister?" said my confused mother.

"I'm your daughter, Sally."

"It gets confusing keeping track of everyone."

"I understand, Mom."

"You've never visited me before." She said, not acknowledging that I had faithfully visited her twice a week for months.

"Maybe you forgot, but I was here last week."

"No, you weren't. What's new with the family?"

We then repeated the same series of questions and answers five times.

"And who are you again?"

The conversation continued in circles. I eventually sat in silence and later left, discouraged and feeling ill equipped to care for my dear mother. Frustrated with my patience being tested, I found myself not always being as gracious as she deserved.

Dementia is a cruel disease that both slowly and rapidly strips people of their dignity without them being aware of it. It strips memories haphazardly. Dementia removes filters and slowly deteriorates the body, although slower than is humane. It turns some people quiet and some become mean. It turns everyone into a different person than who they once strived to be.

There is a period when a person knows something is going wrong. There is a longer period when the family knows that person will never be close to normal again.

A disease of loss and emptiness, dementia is confusing and exhausting. Only death brings freedom, which families are conflicted about saying out loud. Freedom for loved ones brings guilt as it is impossible to do the right things. Dementia has recognizable patterns but a different path for everyone. It brings questions, adjustments, and concessions.

Earth is a broken world and Dementia magnifies the fractures. Our only hope is in the next realm when we know the heavens will open new dimensions with knowledge and God's love.

Drawbridges

Memory pathways in the brain have what I like to describe as drawbridges. Dementia is frequently described as "a bridge went out" between cells — thus causing the loss of the memory of an event or person. However, I see it more as a drawbridge. Memories come and go. Different memories may be scrambled into one. People fill in the blanks with things that did not happen to make sense of the world.

Drawbridges without control become unmanageable and unpredictable. Flexibility and acceptance will help visits become an adventure. Every day will be different, with progress gained and lost.

We spend our lives learning manners and building filters to avoid offending people. Accept that filters are gone so your loved one will say inappropriate things. You may notice uncharacteristic swearing.

This disease is progressive but does not follow a straight path. Memories come and go as your loved one knows you one minute and literally one minute later thinks you are a stranger.

When I visited my mother, she frequently greeted me by name but within five minutes asked who I was. We had nice chats as she asked me if I work, was I married, did I have kids. Pleasant conversation between two polite strangers.

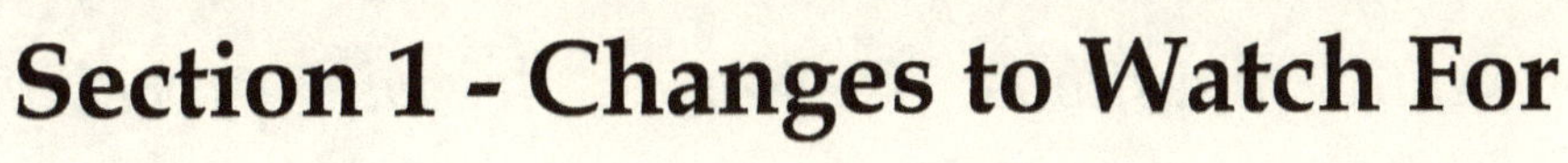

Section 1 - Changes to Watch For

The Beginning

How do you know when dementia begins? You typically do not have a specific point in time that can be identified. It is gradual. It may begin with repeated questions or stories. It will probably include denial, lack of recollection, or aggressiveness. Your loved one snap at you and deny having said something that they clearly had.

Medical events can trigger dementia. Having had anesthesia sometimes increases the confusion for at least some time longer than normally expected. Having a urinary tract infection is also frequently

I think the startling reality for me was when my mom and I were having a conversation and she repeated word for word a question I had just answered. I had her full attention, so it was not just due to multitasking on her part. I also experienced a few instances of her denying I had told her something I clearly had.

Mom was quite the hostess. If you visited, you could be sure she would offer you something to eat. One thing we got used to was being asked 20 times a visit instead of once or twice. "No thanks, Mom. I'm all set."

She had a wall of family pictures in the basement, and every time we visited, we would be escorted down and told who each person was in many pictures.

One of the first things that the family noticed with Mom was confusion about events in the past. Sometimes confusion about family members. I also noticed that she would get increasingly stressed about unfamiliar situations or would easily get lost in a store or mall.

Loss of Skills

Another indicator of oncoming dementia is a loss of once strong physical or dexterity skills. Examples include losing the ability to use a computer, to knit, or to do simple daily tasks. Gradual loss of ability or memory about how to do things is a strong indicator of dementia progressing.

My mom took on computers when she was in her fifties and caught on quickly. She established a website and created a religious booklet with my dad for distribution. After they met in Chicago in the 1950s, the two of them spent their lives in ministry of one form or the other. In their seventies they led a church service weekly at their retirement home. Each week, Dad would preach, and Mom would print Bible verses for his sermon and prepare a CD with songs for the group to sing. Over time, my father noticed she was having trouble printing verses for him. She then started to have trouble putting a CD together each week. He helped her more and more until she no longer knew how to press play on the CD player at the service.

Mom and I regularly emailed each other as I was living in different cities or states and traveling frequently. However, one day Dad asked me to set up email for him so we could communicate. Mom had even lost the ability to send and receive email. We set Dad up on his tablet and shut down her computer for the last time. She did not seem to notice.

Inability to Follow Instructions

Losing the ability to follow simple instructions or to understand cause and effect. We can understand a bit of discomfort to get our teeth cleaned or a needle prick for blood tests. Someone with dementia may not comprehend or tolerate the discomfort.

With the progression of my mother's dementia, we switched her medical care to emergency only. She was so stressed about any appointment that it was difficult to get her to them. Taking her into a lab was almost a major feat. My father would drive her to the building and pled with her to get out of the car. She would finally go in but cry when approached with needles and scream in pain when poked. Nurses were always kind and empathetic but could do nothing to calm her.

We talked to the doctors about calming her with medication. We were able to get low doses of anti-depressants for her but were told that anything more would be considered chemical restraints which are not allowed. We were told anything more sedating would violate her rights.

When her dementia was advanced there was no compliance with directions. She had a heart attack and was bedridden, with no recollection of her heart attack. She didn't have the strength to get out of bed. We took turns caring for her, but in one quick moment she jumped up and scurried across the room and fell, breaking her hip. I have no idea where that burst of energy came from.

Within an hour she was in the hospital for x-rays with no recollection of breaking her hip. She repeatedly asked where she was and why. The doctors confirmed the break and sent us home to call hospice.

In the following days when she would move her hip and feel pain, she was surprised when we explained that her hip was broken. Within a couple of weeks, she was mercifully released from her earthly body.

Changes to Demeanour

Dementia generally changes a person into either a sweeter or meaner person. The change can be shocking.

Mom was always kind. She did not judge strangers and she was generous. However, as dementia ravaged her brain, she became short tempered and downright mean. It was shocking, and I cannot tell you how often I repeated to myself, "The words are coming out of my mother's mouth, but it is the disease that's speaking."

She did not hold back her feelings of resentment for any challenge to her perception of situations. One time I spent the night at my parents' house to see how things were going. Throughout the day and evening, she was aware I was going to stay the night. In the morning, my father and I were up before her. We were sitting in the living room chatting and Mom came into the room in her pajamas and was startled to see me. She marched over to my father and towered over him with her tiny 5-foot frame as he sat in a chair. "Fred, you didn't tell me we were having people stay overnight."

Dad tried to calm her by explaining that she had known, and I had been there the previous day. "Isn't it nice that our daughter came to visit?"

"You did not tell me! Nobody told me people would be staying here in the house! Don't you do that again."

I also tried to diffuse the situation by entering the conversation. "Mom, it's me, Sally. I just wanted to visit my parents."

She did not respond in any way but stood staring at my father.

I repeated myself, a bit louder as she was hard of hearing (although she never admitted it).

Eventually, she spun around and sharply corrected me, "You don't have to repeat yourself. Do not call me Mom! I am not your mother and do not have kids!'

I started to try to calm her and told her she

was my mom. However, she marched over to me and continued to repeat herself, telling me she had no kids and would know if she did.

I threw up my hands in defeat and nodded. "Okay."

She scurried down the hallway in disgust. When she reemerged later, she had a better temperament.

Progression of Sundown Syndrome

One big symptom of dementia is called Sundowning. I am aware of cases where police were called due to extreme confusion. Sundowning brings an increase in confusion over the course of the evening each day. Something clear in the morning becomes the source of confusion and denial when evening arrives. As evening progresses, confusion increases. Obsessive behaviors may increase. Behavior escalates to the point of being frantic. I have heard of people becoming energized and excited but more often it is a negative behavior that is witnessed.

My father had his hands full with my mother in the evening. One trick he would try if she got wound up is to put his coat on. She would ask where he was going. He would tell her they needed to go to the doctor because she was out of control. Fortunately, the threat broke her mood, and she would agree to cooperate and settle down.

At bedtime she would insist she did not know him and would ask where he was sleeping. He would explain that they were married and even show her their marriage certificate. Sometimes it would settle her and other times she would challenge the certificate's authenticity. If she got too agitated, he would start to put his coat on. She would again ask where he was going, and he would offer to sleep in the car. She would soften and offer the twin bed next to hers and they would go to bed.

Mom always loved chocolate. However, as she reached higher and higher levels of insanity through sundowners, she became like a drug addict searching the cupboards for candy. Dad would hide the stash and meter her consumption. If he did not, she would eat an entire bag of candy.

Deterioration of Social Skills

"It's the disease, not the person" is a mantra you may want to repeat to yourself. The disease changes the personality of people with dementia. Accept that filters regarding acceptable behavior and speech are gone. Do not be hurt by anything they say. The words come out of their mouth, but not their heart. They are no longer the same person. The disease is causing mental pain.

My mother lost her filters. She had always been kind and gentle. It was shocking to experience her first signs of dementia which included comments about strangers or judgement of those around her.

Another missing filter was her basic social behavior. My father reached a point where we had to come "babysit" mom if he had an appointment. He had gone to the dentist and could not get Mom to stay in the waiting room. She kept entering the treatment area and even sat in the dentist's chair at one point. It was not unusual for her to approach a receptionist while Dad was in with a doctor. She would ask if the receptionist knew where "the man she came with had gone."

Once we brought a computer with us to Skype with my daughter who was living in a different country. Mom was confused when she looked at the computer screen and saw her own reflection. "Who is that old woman?"

When we told her it reflected herself, she said, "That is not me! I'm not that old." She paced the room and returned to her familiar chair and sat down.

One year, at a family holiday dinner, my daughter and nephew were shocked when my mom abruptly stuck her hands in a punch bowl to break up sherbet that was in lumps larger than she liked. She had made punch for years, but the act of putting bare hands in the full bowl was something that even seemed to catch herself off guard. As the story was told to me, she stood there with orange punch dripping from her hands, not knowing what to do and wondering how she had gotten there.

One last story on this topic. When Mom's

dementia was advanced, she had a heart attack and was hospitalized. My adult nephew came to visit her and brought her a little stuffed hedgehog from the hospital gift shop. She had always loved little stuffed animals.

He brought it in and said, "Here, Grandma, I thought you might like this little guy."

Mom barely had it in her hand and flung it across the room, "I don't want that stupid thing."

Always good natured, he picked it up from the floor and said, "Ok, I guess I'll keep it." And we passed the little guy around the room. We didn't want Mr. Hedgehog to feel rejected.

It is important to have a sense of humor about dementia. Even though it is tragic, it does bring funny moments. We have really laughed a lot about that silly little hedgehog since that incident.

Repetition of Tasks and Speech

Many people with dementia find comfort in repetition. Part of it is not remembering if they did something so they recheck it. Part of it is a need to be busy. Some people get jigsaw puzzles. One person would dump laundry on the bed for repeated folding by her mother. Questions will be repeated over and over with absolutely no recognition the discussion was just had. Keep answering questions with short and vague answers. You will be less frustrated than if you spend ten minutes answering a question that will just be asked again immediately.

In addition to obsessing about ensuring that the doors were all locked, my mother obsessed about trash for some reason. For some reason, all trash had to be in tiny pieces wrapped in masking tape. Inside the trash can, there were smaller containers that contained different types of trash. I usually messed up the entire system when I visited by haphazardly tossing things loosely into the trash can. Yea, I know. Often, I would put some trash into my bag to take home with me to minimize issues.

Dad had told me she was doing poorly in the evening. Having done some research, I learned a lot about sundowner's syndrome, periods of increased agitation often taking place in the evening. I went to stay at my parent's home for a night to see how things were going with Mom.

After an afternoon of Mom worrying about where each person would sleep, I went to bed in the guest room and settled in. Outside the door, my mom kept passing by the door. She would walk from their bedroom to the kitchen to recheck everything and to evaluate each piece of garbage in the trash can. She would take each little piece of trash back to the bedroom to ask my father if it was ok for it to be in the trash can. Dad would patiently tell her that it was ok. After a few passes by my door, I started to count. I counted over 28 round trips before she settled down and went to bed.

On another day, my brother was staying with Mom while Dad went to a doctor appointment. He parked his work truck out front of their home on the street. He brought some paperwork for work he needed to catch up on and sat at the kitchen table working on it.

Mom asked, "Is that paperwork about me? What are you doing?"

Al answered that it was just paperwork he needed to catch up on for work. He offered to show her and talked randomly about his job to make her more comfortable.

She then asked if it was his truck out front. She pointed out that it was blocking the sidewalk.

He explained to her that he had checked with the neighborhood manager to be sure he was parked properly. He had not but felt she would accept it if sounded official.

She seemed ok, but suddenly scurried out the door. She went out to the sidewalk to check his truck. He followed and brought her back in, reassuring her it was ok. She agreed after checking everything out.

She then asked why he was there and where her husband was. He explained that Dad was out for a short time and he was just hanging out to get caught up on paperwork. She scolded him and emphasized she did not need a babysitter.

Finally, she sat down and seemed calmer. Not five minutes later, she was up again to repeat the entire conversation.

She would frequently ask where Dad was when I stayed with her for only a couple hours. She would repeatedly go to the window to see if he was home yet. She would worry that he had been gone all day. "No, Mom. He has only been gone an hour. Let's visit until he gets home."

Hallucinations and Confusion

As part of the process of the brain deteriorating, your loved one may experience hallucinations and confusion about reality. Do not be alarmed, and just listen unless you feel that there is a risk of harm to someone.

Before we moved my mother into a memory care facility, she and Dad lived in a small home in a quiet neighborhood. She spent a lot of time looking out the windows, worrying about things in the area. Mom became overly concerned because fall leaves were blowing onto the neighbors' yards, which she was convinced they were upset about. She was sure there was writing on the leaves about my parents and people might know their business. When it finally snowed, Dad was relieved because all the leaves were covered.

However, she then became concerned when she saw a patch in the driveway without snow on it if the rest of the driveway still had snow. She could not handle the inconsistency of a patchy driveway. The relentless surveillance and paranoia were very wearing on my father.

Whether she was hallucinating or obsessing I do not know, but it was strange behavior that was a challenge.

Obsessive Behaviors

Your loved one may become obsessive about items or behaviors. This is similar to repetition of tasks but can differ as it is an irrational preoccupation with something.

My mother was obsessed with wrapping each piece of garbage with masking tape. Each item was folded as much as possible and then secured with tape.

Shortly after she moved into memory care, I noticed my dad had brought her a role of tape. When I saw him later, I asked, "Dad! What were you thinking by bringing her a new roll of masking tape? I thought since she didn't have tape, she'd adjust to just throwing things away."

"She likes taping her garbage, and she was using band aids. It was cheaper to take her a roll of tape."

I laughed. Yep, a better solution. Until the day she died, she was wrapping her trash with tape.

Because of her obsession with garbage, I would take any of my trash into the hall and dispose in a public bin. One day, I ate a couple of small candy bars and put the wrappers in my pocket. When we went for a walk later, I subtly put them in a hallway trash bin.

On our next loop around the hallway, I could not believe it when she opened that exact trash bin. She was worried when she noticed the wrappers were in there. I challenged her that it might not be our trash – there are other people who also eat that brand of candy. She wasn't convinced, but I did get her to walk away without digging into the bin.

Wandering

Your loved one may wander and even get lost. This can be caused by confusion or excess energy. It can be particularly dangerous if they wander in public or drive away in a car.

My mother gave up driving when her dementia was reaching the mild stage. My father was in the hospital for one night and we never did know what happened exactly. However, my mother took a long time to arrive at the hospital to pick Dad up. She said she got confused getting home the previous evening and getting back in the morning. She never shared, but also never drove again. We appreciated that she did recognize and was scared by whatever her experience was. On the second day, when my father was released, my sister-in-law drove them home.

My mother walked with my father daily as a regular habit. She had some back and hip issues that limited her mobility though, so they normally didn't walk a great distance. However, as her dementia increased, so did her walking.

My father really noticed the walking because it reached a point where he could no longer keep up with her. So, he put two lawn chairs in the front yard – which he said she never used hers. She would walk up and down the street for hours in the late afternoon.

One day, he noticed that she disappeared

from his sight. He sat for a bit and then got worried. He got in the car and drove around the neighborhood for quite some time until he found her. She said she hadn't been lost but he said she seemed panicky and described some places that were quite far from home. He told her to stay on their street from then on.

My family's experiences with wandering were mild compared to many that I've heard. When confused dementia seniors drive away from their familiar settings and disappear for days, silver alerts are triggered. Be on the lookout for this lurking danger.

Section 2 - Cultivating a Comfortable Environment

Simplification of Surroundings

Every family has various approaches to discussing life issues. However, no matter the approach used in the past, keeping it simple is the best approach now. If you are questioned, give short and simple answers. If you decide to get into detail, recognize you will have to repeat yourself in five minutes. You may get an argument with agitation because you are wrong and your loved one has a different perspective. Do not expect to have a deep conversation. Be ready to divert the conversation to wall color if necessary, to keep from going down a rabbit hole of unanswerable questions.

It is also good to simplify the environment by limiting the amount of "stuff" in the home. It can help limit the frequency of things from being lost or obsessed over.

Prior to moving Mom into memory care, Dad got rid of a lot of stuff in their home. He would have to sneak it out, so she wouldn't worry about where it should be or who it belonged to. He donated or gave away furniture, knickknacks and any clutter. He kept the house organized so that he could tell her from his chair which cupboard something was in that she couldn't find. "Are you standing in front of the stove? It is in the cupboard to your right." Otherwise, he would be getting up and down constantly to help her find things that she had just had two minutes ago.

He kept things she loved including a little box with her sisters' things and a nativity scene she repeatedly pointed out to visitors. It was in the living room year-round.

Sticky Notes are Helpful

Use sticky notes as reminders around the house on calendars, doors, and cupboards. It can help remind your loved one what day it is or what time you will be going somewhere that day.

Dad found that Mom would obsess about the calendar and details. For years they had kept a calendar in the kitchen filled with information about appointments and other plans. But this much information became overwhelming for her. Something had to change. So, he left a calendar on the kitchen wall as they had for years, however, it was blank except for one sticky note per day. On a Monday, he would put a sticky note on that day's date that said "Monday", and on each subsequent day he would repeat. He had a little box with stickies for each day of the week.

If they were going somewhere on a particular day, he would put a note on the corner of the counter that day that said, "leaving for lunch at 11:00." It would not eliminate all questions, but if she asked, he could direct her to the note on the counter.

A sticky note might help on a cupboard for dishes or cups. Sometimes it is a retained memory and sometimes it gets confusing about where things are. Just remember to use notes as reminders if they help to simplify things around the house.

Reliving the Deaths of Loved Ones

When they ask about a family member or friend who has been dead for a while, keep in mind that they may have no memory of that loss. Tell them they are busy and will see them soon. Spare them a new round of grief.

Every night at bedtime, my mother would ask my father a series of questions. Many were about him and who he was, but many were about her family. For quite some time, he would go through the list of family members and explain to her they were now dead. She would ask details and be upset and grieve the loss. Eventually, he shortened the nightly monologue to only explain they were not around, but she would be seeing them soon. He did not clarify that, because of their shared Christian religion, he was not lying. We believe we will see family members after death.

Memory Care Decisions

The decision to move a loved one into memory care is heartbreaking. But keeping a person with dementia in their home can be absolutely exhausting for the caregiver(s) and reaches a point that may not be safe. Regardless of your decision, do not allow yourself to second guess your decision or feel guilty. Maybe years ago, your loved one said they would never want to be "put away" but a time may come when the family is unable to provide the care they need and moving them to a facility is necessary.

There is no right or wrong answer!

My family pulled off a well-orchestrated plan when the decision had been made to move Mom into memory care. We told her nothing because she would have disagreed vehemently. Dad took her out for a visit to the mall for a couple hours. My brother, nephew, and I packed up her things and set up her little room at her new facility. It was lovely. We had her familiar furniture and an elaborate setup of family pictures on built-in shelves reaching the ceiling.

After we texted Dad about the room being ready, he brought her into the room. Initially she was confused but quickly changed to being livid. The unpredictable drawbridges in her brain flipped around leaving her seemingly coherent. She was terribly upset and felt betrayed. Following the advice of the staff we did not stay long.

The next day we returned to find all her pictures had been stacked on the sofa ready to return home. She had climbed the shelves and pulled down all the pictures. She was different that day. Instead of anger, she was emotional - which was harder for us to be honest. She was begging my Dad to take her home. I did lose it for a moment and had to leave the room.

There were days when she seemed to be settling in. She did not remember how she got there - seemed to think she just disappeared and showed up in the new place. "They brought me here" - so she already forgot her family ganged up on her and "dumped" her.

Other days she did hold all of us

responsible and kept reminding us of our betrayal. My dad was talented at avoiding questions and answering with non-answers. He kept emphasizing that this is what is best for THEM - the two of them. He used "we" a lot more than "you" when talking to her. She repeatedly asked how long - and he said, "we're still evaluating". She repeatedly asked how much money it cost, and he would tell her "it's complicated - I haven't sat down and figured that out yet."

I brought in a journal I left in her drawer so we could write the date and a note whenever we visited. Although I have read some families have found success, in our case, it was not helpful. She did not believe what was written and still insisted we never visited. She had been surrounded by pictures of her family, but now they permanently resided in a dresser drawer.

Even though my Dad would leave every day, she thought he was living there too because she would talk about "we live here now but I don't like it."

Mom lived there for five months. At the end of five months my father felt he wanted to take care of her again. It was difficult for him to visit her every day feeling helpless to do anything. So, we researched assisted living facilities and we moved them into a lovely place near us. Assisted living provided more care than he needed and less than she needed. He was able to provide care, with the help of assisted living care, that was sufficient when he could no longer provide all care by himself.

The Meaning of Home

When most people with dementia say they want to go home, they are seeking a place of less confusion and more comfort. They are living in a state of confusion and want to return to what they frequently picture as their childhood home, not the house they just left. It also means they are looking for a life slipped away. So, when you visit, you may be faced with repeated pleas to take them home. However, you must recognize "home" is no longer an option, but a point and place in the past that cannot be returned to.

Understand your loved one is now living in the past,

remember there are years haphazardly missing from memory. People will be mixed up through the wrong memories. I found asking about their young years will frequently bring more memories than anything recent.

My mother frequently asked to go home. I had learned of this phenomenon among people with dementia, so I tried different things. I asked her to describe home or would use the diversion tactics to suggest we would be going home soon.

One day when Mom had been in memory care for several months, complaining daily about it. Dad had decided to move her to an assisted living location where he would live with her.

My brother and I arrived one day and explained to her with excitement we would be moving her out that day. We were expecting to be greeted with glee that we were finally getting her out of the "hellhole" as she called it.

However, she sat on her couch with her arms crossed and said, "I don't want to move. I never thought this place was bad. It's a nice place."

My brother and I looked at each other. Just like move-in day, we had Dad take her out and drive to their new place that was all ready for them. We loaded up her stuff and headed out.

After we moved Mom into assisted living, back with Dad, she settled down. She never had any memory of being in Memory care for five months. Her obsessive behavior continued but being back with my father seemed to return her to a sense of "home."

Once they were back together, she seemed more settled, but she did ask my father repeatedly when they would be moving home.

Section 3 - Tips for Visiting

Talk a Lot and Delay

You may want to plan for a few things you can just ramble about. Talk in detail about your day. Talk in detail about the ingredients you put into a recipe or the details of a tv show you recently watched. Accept you probably will not have a conversation but can fill silence with simple stories. Do not expect there will be any recollection.

Confusion can lead to frustration. If your loved one gets stuck on something, suggest it can be sorted out later. "We'll figure that out tomorrow. Let us not worry about it today."

When I visited my mother, I would tell her stories about my dogs. Other times I talked about somewhere I traveled – maybe an unusual custom I experienced in different countries.

If she asked when she was going to be moved back home, I would tell her we would talk to Dad about it soon. I learned to be quite evasive and noncommittal.

I frequently redirected our conversations. My mother used to love to talk about her childhood. I would ask her about the house she lived in as a child. I cannot tell you how many times she told me about sledding on the snowy street in front of her house in Maine. If I could get her started down that path, she would talk for some time.

Logic Comprehension

Do not expect an understanding of logic. A person with dementia does not understand they are sick and need help. There may be rare, fleeting moments of awareness that something is going wrong.

Mom had moments when she asked my father what was going wrong with her. She expressed appreciation to him for taking care of her. She knew that something was wrong but did not understand. Within a minute she would snap back into dementia with no recollection of her moment of clarity. Those brief moments of understanding gave him strength and hope to get through the rest of the caregiving challenges.

Once we had moved Mom into memory care, I felt I was failing at being a supportive daughter when visiting. My mother constantly asked how she got into a memory care facility of all places given she had no problems with her memory. She repeatedly asked who put her there and what she had done wrong. As a family, we strived for consistency with "you need help with your memory"; "the doctor felt this was best for you". However, she was not a sweet little old lady like I know she would have wished to be. She was quite nasty. "There's nothing wrong with my memory." "I've always taken care of family, who has now dumped me in here like a dirty little monkey."

One day I tried to explain she had become unsafe in her home with Dad because at night she did not recognize him and was fearful. She was threatening to kick him out of her home. Of course, as expected, she denied it and got angry. I cried and she scowled.

Mom's memory at that point was about thirty seconds long - two minutes tops. So, after my grand attempt to explain the situation honestly, she looped back to her first question. I learned to keep things simple, "It's what's best for you right now, Mom."

Let Them Lead Visits

Every day will be different. One day you might find a somewhat cheerful person who you can chat with about fun memories. Other days you may find someone sleeping in their chair. Take a bit of time when arriving to determine the mood of the day. Allow your loved one to decide if you walk the halls or sit still. Allow the conversation to go where they lead. Use your skill in distraction to change directions as needed.

Sometimes my mom would be in her chair napping when I visited. She did not want to go for a walk. Other times she wanted to walk the halls of her memory care and point out things in activity tables around the home.

Every time my brother visited; she would repeat a story about his childhood. She had changed the details, but Al just nodded and agreed. We lived on a farm with a tall silo. My brother climbed the ladder to the top and took pictures we had through the years giving us a great perspective from the air.

However, whenever Mom told the story, it included him climbing up on the top and walking around the edge. That did not happen, but it was somehow created in her memories and became as entrenched as the real memories of the climb and pictures.

I also learned through my visit to have

patience with detail. One day I took her a nightstand. I did not put it in the right spot. She rearranged and was happy. Honestly, I could not see a difference between my placement versus hers. But she was happy and probably adjusted it twenty times throughout the day.

Learn to Stretch the Truth

Do not think of skirting the truth as lying. If it bothers you, skip answering a direct question with a diversion.

My father told me after being married for sixty-five years of trying not to lie to his wife he had to become a liar. It was good for limiting arguments and to stop agitation. Mom would get very anxious about upcoming events, so he started to keep a secret calendar and put nothing on the kitchen wall calendar. He would tell her about any appointments just before they had to leave for it.

After years of being dressed impeccably, my mother became resistant to change. She wore a terribly worn wig. She had socks with holes in them and her clothing was well worn. One day I gave the nurses a new wig, socks, and bras for my mother. I knew she would not be receptive to anything I gave her, so I conspired with the nurses. When they gave her a bath, they made the old wig disappear and gave her the new one. She was not happy but was wearing it the next day. It looked great and I found forgiveness for myself for the lies. She forgot the old one before I did.

Shortly after the plot to switch out her things, she told me people were taking her things. Like her wig and socks, which left her with only "these new socks that keep falling down". Oops, I did my best to match the ones she was wearing but could not find socks that exactly matched.

One day Mom asked me if I had brought her the wig she was wearing. I said "no, I didn't. But it looks great!" I became quite skilled at lying.

Mom became obsessed with the cost of things. She had grown up poor and had returned there in her mind. One day we went to an ice cream shop and she saw that ice cream cones were $2.50. She refused to allow me to buy her one because they should only be ten cents. So, I adjusted my approach.

Knowing that if I brought her a sandwich, she would insist on knowing how much it cost.

If I told her five dollars, she would refuse to eat it because I should never have spent that much money on a sandwich. So, I learned to lie and tell her it was one dollar. She would then eat the sandwich and love it, going on and on about what a great deal it was at one dollar. Yes, I was lying to her, but it was in defense of her flawed logic as her dementia progressed.

Lose Your Memory

If your loved one claims you are not related, just say ok. If they tell you something is not theirs, just say ok. If a person with dementia argues that you are not telling them the truth just say ok. Another approach is to act just as stumped as the loved one and say, "We will just have to look into that."

It is a good idea to lose your memory. If you cannot recall details, then you will avoid an argument. "I'm sorry, I can't remember those details anymore."

One day Mom asked who I was and who Dad was. We explained and she was pleased to hear that I am Sally - her daughter.

Not two minutes later she asked who we were again. We explained, but she denied I was her daughter.

However, Dad did claim me. Mom then got upset and talked about how overwhelming all this information was to her. She was having trouble processing how her husband had a daughter with another woman (so evidently, she did remember who he is).

She asked me what my mother's name is. I said Molly. She said she is NOT my mother. I said "well, are you the only Molly in the world?" (yea, I know I was a bit argumentative - it slipped)

She then said she KNOWS her children and I am NOT one of them. I asked who her children were, and she told me she did not have to tell me.

Dad told her she needs to be polite to me since it was nice of me to visit every day. She said she would but pointed out I had never been there before.

I asked her if it was ok to visit with my dad. She said yes, but she felt all this information crashing down on her. She wanted to know what we were all going to do about this. Dad asked what she would like to do about it. He told her they would sort out all the paperwork about it later - and that seemed to calm her. He got a folder out and started shuffling papers.

He was talented at coming up with off the wall stuff to calm her. I had to stop myself from laughing (if I laughed too much, she accused me of laughing at her). Paperwork? Really? Paperwork is going to sort out this confusion of her husband having a daughter with someone else.

Externally I maintained a straight face. However, internally I was crying while also laughing that we were sitting there experiencing this. At 60 years of age, I had to identify my mother - to my mother!

Visiting with Children

Recognize that even if your loved one always adored children, their behavior may cause unpredictable problems. I recommend caution when bringing children to visit a person with dementia. Sometimes the behavior shifts can cause coarse language and a lack of social filters when talking to children.

I went to visit Mom with my 3-year-old grandson. I learned to not visit without a backout plan. She was berating me as usual including a repeated phrase of "you are part of the family who put me in this Hellhole, and I resent it." And she ignored my darling grandson's attempts to talk to her as she cursed in front of him. I had him bring books to read so we would have a quiet visit. He was an angel, by the way - seriously. Bless his heart. However, in the middle of a book, Mom said, "do you have to read books to him here? Can't you do that at home?"

I told her I had him bring books so we could have a pleasant visit. If I was disturbing her, I could leave. She said, "that's up to you - you're the visitor."

"Who's the kid?" "Does he live with you?" "You better keep him with you while here."

Although I had become accustomed to being heartbroken by this insanity, that day took it to a new level. I just did not get why she had to be so mean - and to an adorable 3-year-old. We left after about a half hour. My grandson took it all in stride. I had warned him she would be grumpy. After we left, he told his mom, "She was feeling very grumpy today."

On other days when I visited with my grandsons, my mom was fascinated with them. She might really love a toy that they were playing with and repeatedly comment on it. She would even give them hugs.

It just depended on the day and mood. I tried to gauge the situation when I arrived and have an escape plan if it looked questionable.

Popular Topics

For many, a deep belief in God does not leave. At times, diverting agitation to talk of the afterlife can be calming. Urge your loved one to discuss the details of an experience they had at some point in their life. Just let them talk, encouraged with a few short questions. This can be applied to any topic they seem to find joy in discussing.

Identify a topic that is specific to the person - military service, career, or hobbies. Some people spent a lot of time traveling. What is important is to try to find a topic that elicits passion.

Because my mom was Christian, she loved her Bible. It always sat beside her on a little table. I would try to get her to talk by asking questions about the Bible or heaven. I would ask her what her favorite verse was. I asked what she thought Heaven would look like. Sometimes it would perk her up and get her talking. Other times she would not, but it gave me something to ask her about.

She loved to tell me about a gospel singer she liked. It was sad for me to watch as she would hold her cd player in her lap and wonder why it was not playing. However, she was no longer able to understand the concept of headphones. So, I just listened as she talked about various songs.

As a young woman she took a train from

Maine to Chicago to attend Moody Bible Institute with little money but a large amount of passion for Jesus. She had a passion for children's ministry. She lit up when I would ask her about driving a big school bus for a kid's program that she ran. Those topics would sometimes get her talking.

Silence

It is perfectly acceptable to sit in silence during visits. This is not the time to correct their version of events or to have deep conversations. Just keeping someone company can sometimes be enough without words.

Somedays I would visit Mom and she would be sleeping in her chair. I would quietly slip in the room and just sit until she awoke. Other times we went outside in the secured patio area for residents. We probably sat for thirty minutes to an hour without saying anything. It was a challenge for me, but I learned something from it.

She would take things in and out of her purse the entire time we sat on a bench in the garden. She was puzzled by why a small flashlight didn't work. After suggesting she needed new batteries a few times, I learned to be quiet. The activity of taking the flashlight apart and reassembling was an activity that seemed to satisfy her.

I did not recognize how poor Mom had become with general conversation until she was in memory care. I realized that for years, when I visited my parents it was pretty much my father who I had conversations with. When it was just me visiting Mom in memory care, I recognized that it was me who had to carry what communication we did have. It felt quite

awkward until I recognized it for what it was.

Me, filling a void of silence.

Abrupt Change

Recognize that taking someone out of their familiar setting may not lead to the enjoyable break you may expect – even if they are asking for it. When determining whether an outing for lunch or family gatherings is a good idea, take small cautious steps. Consider leaving your loved one in their familiar safe environment as it may be better for them.

When I was a kid, my parents used to take us on Sunday drives through the countryside. We would drive aimlessly and perhaps stop for a candy bar along the way. After I grew up and moved on, my parents continued the habit.

My mother loved going for car rides and they had their routines of driving somewhere on the weekend and stopping for lunch. However, as my mother developed dementia my father started to shorten the drives. She would become distraught and confused as they drove around. She would cry and ask where they were. It was easier to stay home than to deal with her stress and confusion.

For years they went go to the grocery store a couple times a week and split up to each do their own thing. Each would shop for whatever they needed and meet at the front of the store. Over time, my mother started to become anxious and confused. She was paranoid that people were trying to steal her purse – which may or may not have been true. My father reached a point where he had to keep her with him while shopping. She would still be stressed but felt safer with him. She followed him as he made all the buying decisions for them. She no longer cared or understood. She might say she needed something, perhaps socks, when they were home. However, she would panic at the store and deny needing them and refuse to even go into that department.

One day I got a new car and Dad wanted a ride, which was typical when any of us had a new vehicle. So, I picked my parents up and drove around a large block in nearby countryside. Mom cried for the entire ten-minute drive - wondering where we were going. We then parked back in their driveway and I walked into their apartment to visit for a while. That small jaunt in a strange car threw her off bringing her sundowners on earlier that day. She was also confused about who I was and why I came into their apartment with them.

Visit Again

Do not stay away. Dementia is a long journey, but sadly does end. Over time, better memories of your loved one will return. While in the midst of the battle it is sometimes hard to put the whole of a lifetime in perspective.

I regularly visited Mom but was told each time that I had never been there. Mom would greet me as Sally but forget who I was within five minutes. Despite being frustrating, I do not look back and regret visiting.

I do not even regret our final Mother's

Day. I had given my mother flowers every year on Mother's Day and she always loved them. While she was living in memory care, I brought her a vase with a simple arrangement of light and dark pink carnations with baby's breath. I cheerfully greeted her, "Hi Mom, I brought you some flowers for Mother's Day!"

"If you cared, you wouldn't leave me in this prison. I don't want anything from you. You can leave now. And take those flowers with you."

I reassured her I did care and wanted to visit for a while. I tried distraction by asking if I could just leave the flowers there for a day or so but pick them up when I visit again. But no, she was adamant I take them and go. It was another reminder to recognize the disease not the person, but I walked down the hall and out the door with tears in my eye avoiding contact with anyone lest I burst into tears. With sadness I returned home and set the flowers on my dining room table and watched them wilt over the next week or so.

Visits can take sudden turns in unexpected directions. On another visit, after sitting sullenly in the garden, we were returning to her room when another resident tried talking to me. My mother actually turned to the other lady and snapped, "Leave her alone. She is MY daughter."

I was pleased because it showed that somewhere in there, my mother knew who I was.

They know we are visiting. They just

cannot always process things the way we would like. On the rare day that she was cheerful, it would help to make up for the miserable visits.

When on a trip near the end of her life, I wrote a short note to her on hotel stationary and mailed it to her. I didn't hear anything about it but knew she received it from my father. After she died, when I went through her purse, I found a weathered envelope, barely hanging together, tucked into the back pocket. It was the blue envelope with my handwriting on it with my note. She had kept it tucked away and had clearly handled it often, even in her confusion. I still have it.

In Conclusion

The journey of dementia does have a conclusion. It is a tragic end with no resolution. I understand that there are medications that can slow the progression but not stop it. The support of a family is immeasurably helpful to each other as well as to the casualty of dementia.

The end can come slowly as the brain deteriorates, taking away the physical ability to eat and breath. Or another physical ailment may take over ending the journey. For my mother, she had a heart attack, followed by a broken hip. We saw that as a blessing to end her misery.

Each journey is as unique as it is different. I hope that by sharing my story you find tips, hope, and maybe even a chuckle or two. Without humor, life is utterly dismal. My goal is to seek laughter in each day and smile as I recall the good days with my mom. This is incredibly hard - remember to inhale and exhale.

A Tribute to Mom

(September 12, 2018)

This is something I wrote the day after Mom died as my way of closure.

My mother died yesterday. However, I lost my mom a while ago to Alzheimer's disease. I can't really remember exactly when it started. Maybe with a few repeated questions. Maybe a few repeated tasks. Slowly she slipped away and there was nothing we could do about it. Sometimes she knew who we were and other times she didn't. It was terrifying for her as well as the family. Knowing it was a disease didn't ease the pain. My heart broke a little bit more each time she slipped further away. I was frustrated with myself when I lost patience. I was angry that I could do nothing to fix it. I soaked up short moments when she seemed like herself. I reached for her as she retreated into the fog.

If you knew Mom "in her prime", she was a firecracker. She was tiny in stature but had more heart and spirit than giants. She exhausted me with her energy. There was no task too big or daunting for her. And nothing would stop her from sharing her love for Jesus.

I am conflicted as I rejoice with her freedom from earth. I knew the disease would take her life, so it wasn't a shock. Instead, it was honestly a relief. However, as long as she was here and able to step into her well-worn slippers each morning, we didn't have to feel the void that her absence would bring.

Shortly before she left us, she returned to me only briefly. The Alzheimer's journey was truly Hell on earth but was erased momentarily as her frail arms reached for me through layers of morphine. She smiled and said, "I love you." I could tell that it was her.

She was surrounded by the love of many who stood vigil as she endured one setback after another. After two heart attacks and a broken hip, even hospice was puzzled that she hung on. Those of us who knew her were not surprised at her toughness.

I'll miss my mom.

About the Author

Sally Stap is a mother and grandmother. However, it is the experience of being a daughter that led to this journey.

Sally also wrote about her personal Acoustic Neuroma brain tumor experience in the book Smiling Again: Coming Back to Life and Faith After Brain Surgery.

Appendix – Summary of Tips

The Beginning - It is gradual. It may begin with repeated questions or stories. It will probably include denial, lack of recollection or aggressiveness.

Loss of Skills - Understand that many lifelong physical skills will be deteriorated or lost.

Inability to Follow Instructions - Losing the ability to follow simple instructions or to understand cause and effect.

Changes to Demeanor - Dementia may change one's temperament. Some people become mean; others become nice. This is unpredictable and may differ significantly from the personality they had before.

Progression of Sundown Syndrome - As the day progresses, agitation increases causing frustration, confusion, or possibly increased energy as the sun sets.

Deterioration of Social Skills - Social filters of what is appropriate deteriorate. Inappropriate things may be said including cursing.

Repetition of Tasks and Speech - Because the brain is no longer capable of short-term memory, repetition of very short-term experiences or questions becomes common.

Hallucinations and Confusion - As part of the process of the brain deteriorating, your loved one may experience hallucinations and confusion about reality.

Obsessive Behaviors - Because the brain is confused, obsessive behavior is common and visual confusion is frequently experienced.

Wandering - Your loved one may wander and even get lost. This can be caused by confusion or excess energy. It can be particularly dangerous if they wander in public or drive away in a car.

Simplification of Surroundings - Try to eliminate clutter and keep the environment easy to live in so that things cannot be misplaced or fretted about. This may take some effort over time but will make life easier for all.

Sticky Notes are Helpful - Use sticky notes as reminders around the house on calendars, doors or cupboards. It can help remind of what day it is or what time you will be going somewhere that day.

Reliving Death of Loved Ones - The memory of events and deaths is probably sporadic, faded, or gone; so, avoid discussion of who may have died. Instead of reminding them that loved ones have died, try to vaguely discuss that they are not around currently.

Memory Care Decisions - It is hard to make the decision to move another person into an institutional living environment, but it is sometimes the best decision for everyone. Do not feel guilty. Take advantage of anyone you can ask for guidance.

The Meaning of Home - We all have our definition of what home is, but it changes for anyone with dementia. Home becomes an unachievable place in memory that cannot be returned to. Ask questions about what home was like and avoid commitments to return to it.

Talk a Lot and Delay - Conversation with someone with dementia can never be described as deep, so keep things light and try to come up with insignificant things to talk about. Delay discussion of anything that may cause agitation.

Logic Comprehension - Trying to explain things truthfully can cause frustration and agitation at times. Try to simplify. Do not use logic if a person with dementia clearly cannot process logic. Possibly adjust to whatever degree of logic is digestible for the stage the person is in.

Let Them Lead Visits - Mood of the day is the best way to gauge a visit. If sleepy, just sit and be with someone. Walk the halls if desired. Listen if agitated. Be sensitive to and aware of their mood and allow your loved one to lead your visit.

Learn to Stretch the Truth - You may have to adjust your explanations to avoid difficult conversations. Remember that this is sometimes the best way to help your loved one. If you replaced threadbare socks with new ones and your loved one protests, it might be best to deny knowledge of what happened to them.

Lose Your Memory – It is a good idea to lose your memory. If you cannot recall details, then you will avoid an argument.

Visiting with Children - Be aware of the mood of a person with dementia before taking children to visit. It can be a delightful experience and lift spirits for all. However, it can also be stressful and confusing for the children if you visit on a day your loved one is especially negative or confused.

Popular Topics – It is helpful to get someone to talk about something that they have memories about. Perhaps religion, military, hobbies, or travel. What is important is to try to find a topic that elicits passion.

Silence - Just sit with them. This is not the time to correct them or have deep conversations.

Abrupt Change - Recognize taking someone out of their familiar setting may not lead to the enjoyable break you may expect.

Visit Again - Do not stay away. Dementia is a long journey, but sadly does end. The memory of the "real" loved one will take over those of the compromised person overtaken by dementia.

Each journey is as unique as it is different. I hope that by sharing my story you find tips, hope, and maybe even a chuckle or two. Without humor, life is utterly dismal. This is incredibly hard - remember to inhale and exhale.

Acknowledgements

I acknowledge the incredible work family members in our vast world dedicate to those who are compromised by disease.

Thank you, Fred and Molly Stap for being my parents.

Thank you, Kayla and Kendra for being my daughters and listening to my book ideas.